My Life's Journey

My Life's Journey
Copyright © 2011 by Richard J. Cushing
All Rights Reserved
ISBN 1461081939
ISBN 9781461081937

My Life's Journey

by

Richard J. Cushing

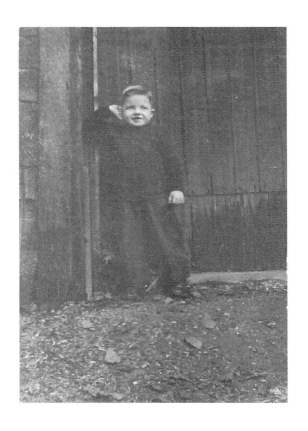

"This book is dedicated to helping others find solutions to their problems no matter how difficult they may seem."

Richard J. Cushing

Hi, my name is Richard J. Cushing
and this is my story....

My life started pretty simple. I was born in Boston Massachusetts and raised in Roxbury. I was lucky I grew up with two brothers, a sister and cousins who lived nearby. We were young, with no problems between us, just love for each other.

We were a poor family but most of the time happy. My brothers and I shared the only bedroom and all slept on the same bed. My sister and mother shared a small bed in a little sunroom and my father slept on the couch in the parlor. Of course we had hard times, but we always stayed close as a family.

Each day began with a vitamin and a tablespoon of cod liver oil because it made you strong. I once jumped off a barn roof when I was 10 years old thinking I was super strong and broke my arm which was a big deal. I never dreamed how minor my injury was compared to now.

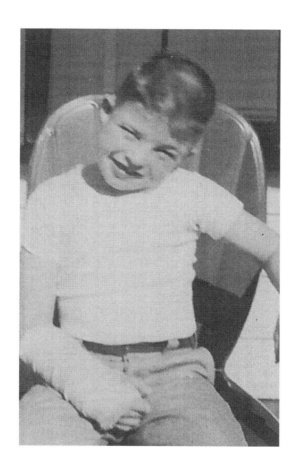

Each day at lunchtime we were allowed to leave school to run home nearby for something to eat. My brothers and I always ate our lunch at Aunt Dottie's house for some reason. It was always a warm feeling there. Mostly we would eat soup with a glass of milk.

Our favorite games were playing cowboys or army. In those days, family meant something; loyalty, honesty and love. My brothers and I along with my cousins were altar boys at Carmel and for the Little Sisters of the Poor who gave us sweet donuts for serving mass. We use to argue over who would light the candles or who rang the bells during mass.

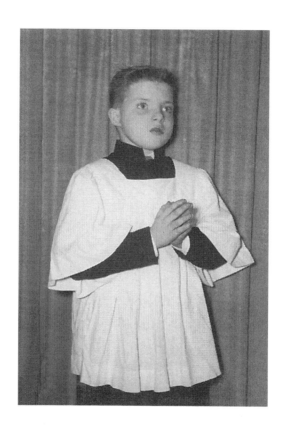

In the old days when I was a kid, you never showed your emotions. You never cried or yelled. If you did, you got the belt. Today kids are given timeouts instead of the belt.

As our neighborhood was becoming more dangerous we knew we had to move. The decision was made and we all packed up and went to Milton. It was like going to another world. I never saw so many trees or heard so much quiet. It took a lot of adjusting not knowing anyone or knowing our way around. Everyone outside of my family who had been close to me were now gone and would only be seen again at birthdays or family get together's.

I never fit in a school as far back as I can remember. Those who didn't know me made fun of me along with some who did know me. This led to fighting which got me in trouble a lot. I didn't pay close attention to my studies which resulted in low grades. I found myself isolated and in need of change.

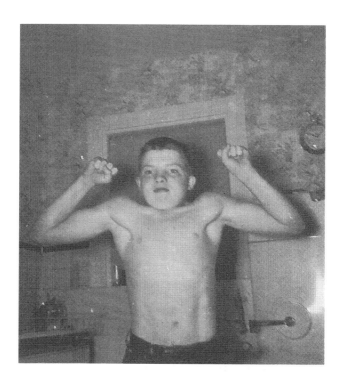

My father thought that taking a job at the New England Phone Co. and finishing school at a later time might be best for me. It made sense because I wasn't learning anything. The year was 1965 when I went to work full time. Each morning my dad gave me 15 minutes to do the essentials and be in the car so he could drive me to work. While in the car he drilled me on things to remember. He reminded me over and over to always be on time, never leave work early and always have a close shave.

Over the years I have always stuck to those simple rules. I started off working in the mail room which I kind of enjoyed. I got to know some of the workers and they invited me to go bowling with them. Pretty soon, I was on a bowling team from work and got to wear a cool team jacket. This was great I thought. I could drink beer and have some laughs with the guy's. Life was good. I felt like a man with money in my pocket. Looking back at school, I grew angry at the way they had treated me but that was behind me now and good riddance.

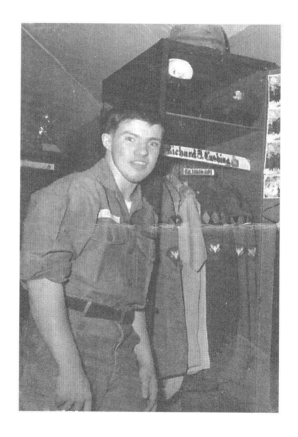

The news papers and television talked about this place called Vietnam and how we were sending soldiers there to fight the bad guys. I began to think that I wanted to be one of the soldiers to go there. I'd now been on the job for a couple of years so the union would hold my job till I came back. I wanted to get away from home and be a man so I joined the U.S. Army. Signing up was a very proud day for me. As a young kid, I always watched army movies and played army with my brothers and cousins. I never thought I would really be there.

When I first entered the service I thought it would be like the John Wayne movies I watched but after getting there, I was sad and it was a rude awakening. I was scared at first but I slowly became ok with it. I was used to being yelled at so that was not anything new. My first day, I complained about something and they made me do fifty pushups. I learned to never complain again. I was assigned to the infantry which meant the possibility of going to Vietnam. Graduation from boot camp was a special day for me and my family. I had never completed anything in my life up to this point. It was the happiest day of my life up till then. My parents came to New Jersey for the ceremony and they too were proud and happy that day.

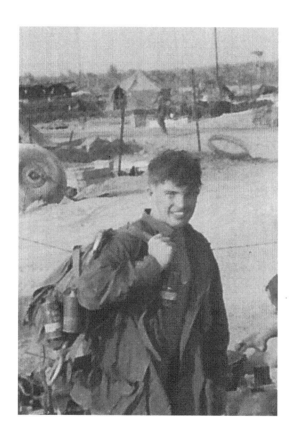

After completing further training I was shipped to Korea which was very cold in the winter. To pass away my free time hours, I would drink to be sociable. The alcohol made me overcome my fears of strangers. Drinking also caused problems. I began to drink while on duty and my performance was less than expected. Rank would come and go depending on my ability to control my bad habits.

After Korea, I received orders for Germany. I thought I would be shipped to Vietnam but I didn't. Instead I received orders to a country known for its beer which sounded good to me. I was hoping to get a fresh start but my bad habits continued to cause me problems with my company's First Sergeant. After being there for six months, I requested duty in Vietnam. It wasn't until almost a year had gone by that my orders for Vietnam came in. Before you're sent to Vietnam, you are given a few weeks off to go home. Life looked very different to me. I saw lots of guy's with long hair and dressed differently than I remembered. My friends took every chance to celebrate my orders for Vietnam by drinking beer together. On the day I left, I was looking out the window of the plane as it took off from Logan Airport wondering if I would ever see home again . It's one thing talking about war and training for it but it's pretty scary when you get orders to actually go.

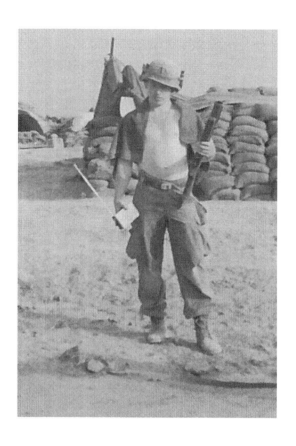

I remember as our jet approached Vietnam in 1968, a pair of jet fighters provided escort. I was assigned to the 1st Calvary Airmobile Infantry division. The First Cav ! I had no idea what was to come during my tour of duty. What made the division special was its ability to travel fast, light and strong in the Huey H1 or Chinook. We weren't always traveling around in helicopters though.. We spent lots of time on base digging and filling sandbags or standing duty at a perimeter fence gates or perimeter towers for 12-15 hours at a time. Most of our free time was spent writing letters, drinking beer or smoking the ganja and tending to foot fungus or jungle rot. Whatever kept you going, you did quietly. We also had outside patrols.

My first experience of war came just before the dawn of a star filled night. A huge whumping sound made everything seem to shake and red flashes with a dark smoke seemed to be all over. During this chaos, I kept my head down behind a wall of sandbags, hoping that nothing would land in my area. I can remember gritting my teeth and holding my M16 as tight as I could. I was both terrified and shocked and after what seemed like forever, the noise and shaking stopped. I learned that we had been attacked by a dozen or so rockets which only actually lasted minutes.

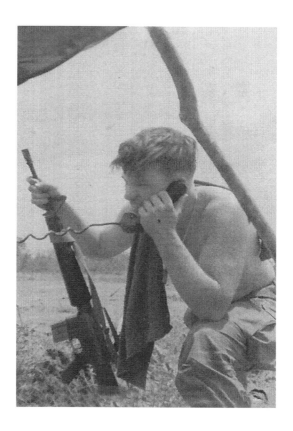

Immediately following the barrage, everyone was on the perimeter at maximum alert for the next few hours in the event of a ground attack. The fear that overwhelmed us was soon turned into laughter and brave talk about how we were gonna kick their ass for what they did to us. We were the First Cav. Bad move Charlie! I was feeling better.

I experienced other moments of war which I survived and each one took its toll on my nerves. There are more war stories to tell but this book is not about the war in Vietnam. It's about a war I hadn't fought yet, one that I would have to fight myself, my war with Parkinson's.

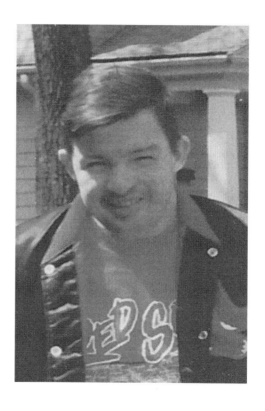

Any sort of loud noise makes me jumpy. It is very scary being in a war never knowing what's going to happen next and where it is going to come from. Rockets do that to you. As a member of the infantry, I was proud to have earned the Combat Infantry Badge during my tour of duty there which recognizes multiple engagements with the enemy. I no longer felt I needed to prove myself to anyone.

I departed Vietnam after an extended tour and after serving a few months of state side duty, I received an Honorable Discharge from the U.S. Army. My younger brother would also serve in Vietnam. I met him at the airport when he returned and was so happy to see him safely home again. I was very proud of him as a brother and as a fellow soldier.

Civilian life was not an easy transition. When I first came home from Vietnam, I felt uneasy and overwhelmed. You can't just turn the soldier off and civilian switch on. Simple pleasures like a private bathroom, a real bed or driving in a car were like first time experiences. Not carrying or needing your weapon(s) by your side also took a little time to get used to. I continue to feel jumpy around loud noises and my right hand will still clinch shut from time to time. I thought that in time these things would take care of themselves. Time passed but the symptoms were not getting any better. In fact, things were probably getting worse. Remember the rules, no complaining.

To deal with these issue's, I did what I always did to take the pain away, I drank and then drank some more until everything was ok. As the next few years passed, my drinking was putting my job in jeopardy. I was showing up at the wrong time or not showing up at all. I would sometimes sleep in a company truck parked in the garage during working hours working off a hangover. Friend's would try to cover up for me but eventually word would reach my father of his son's work record.

He was the one who helped getting me my job with instructions to show up and be on time. It was a major embarrassment to him because he was a supervisor. The whole repair group reported to him. If not for my dad and the effort's of telephone workers union, I might have lost my job long ago.

A couple of reps I'll always be especially grateful to are Fitzy and Myles who put themselves at risk by trying to help straighten out my life and my job. I owe them a lot. My father helped get me a new position internally where I would be more accountable. He warned me that he was not going to be able to save my job if I screwed up another time. With no truck to sleep in anymore or lunches drinking beer, things were going to hopefully be better for me or so I thought.

One night I went to McDonalds to buy my dinner and at the counter I was greeted by a beautiful smile and a friendly hello. Her name tag said Debbie. Smiling back at her, I forgot what I was going to order. I was only thinking about how to get to know her. I laughingly ordered some food and paid her. While I was waiting for my order I could not stop looking at her and as I was leaving she waved goodbye to me.

I was feeling real good. Should I ask her out on a date I thought? I did not want to seem anxious so I waited a day before returning at the same previous time and she was there. This time I introduced myself and suggested we meet after her work. Holding my breath she smiled and said, yes. I dated Debbie for a year and we eloped in New Hampshire. I was happy as hell and life was good.

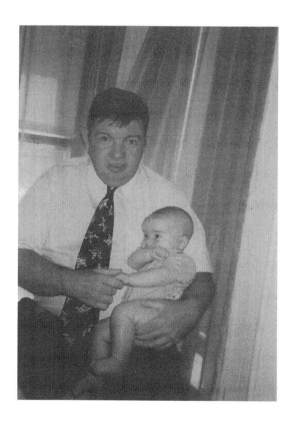

In the beginning, she put up with my drinking and card playing with the boys but once she got pregnant, she wanted me to stop everything. I assured her that I would cut down on my drinking and limit myself to just having a few and quitting gambling. Betting on football, baseball and horses would no longer be a problem or so I thought.

Not long after, the most beautiful day in my life happened. I was a father to a beautiful baby girl. We named her Belinda after her grandmother. I was never so happy. We were a proud young couple settling down with a family.

The economy was weakening and the phone company was in hard times, so all overtime would be eliminated. I tried gambling to make up for the lost wages using a local bookie. My luck was not very good and the losses began mounting, so I used my credit cards to feed my betting. Because of the pressures I began drinking most of everyday.

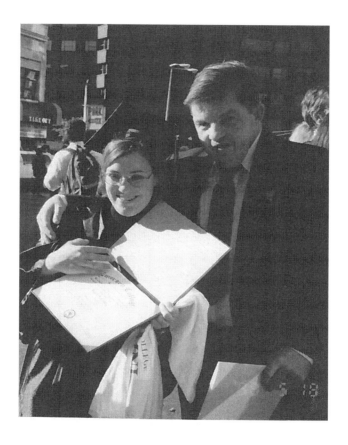

The credit cards let me fool my wife but after maxing out my credit cards, I had to take a loan from the telephone credit union which for awhile kept my credit cards up to date and my wife thinking all was ok. In the end it all fell apart. I was in debt for some thirty thousand dollars. I recall the yelling and crying and awful words exchanged to each other. I had let down my family and I would spend the rest of my life trying to make it up in some way to my daughter. She was everything to me. This was no life for a family with a young child.

We separated with Belinda going with her mother and I moved back to my parent's home, broke, ashamed, in debt and shaken by all that had happened. I spent the next few years trying hard to get my life back together but when you fall as far as I did, it takes a lot of time to climb back up.

Just before Belinda was entering her 7th grade, her mother came to our house to discuss Belinda's future. She did not feel that she could adequately care for her any longer and that I needed to retain custody of her. I was completely shocked and did not know how to respond. My parents had already raised seven kids and were entering their retirement years but my parents loved Belinda and took her in to care for her.

Belinda and I were very, very fortunate and thankful to this day. Through the love of a large family, a potential tragedy was averted. Having Belinda with me gave me the chance to be with her much more and one of our favorite activities was bowling. We joined a father/daughter team and were the champions for a couple of years. Belinda and I shared a special song named "I just called to say, I love you". We had some wonderful times together which I hoped would make up in some way my failures as a father earlier in her life.

Looking back at my situation, I realized how much damage my drinking caused my wife and child and my own family as well. While I could not do anything about the past, I could try to change my future. My all time best friend OB helped me with my work and drinking problems and was always there to help me during the good times and the bad. He has since passed on but not in my heart.

I stopped drinking in 1983, when I joined Alcoholics Anonymous. It was here that I met a lot of people with the same problem who understood the illness and offered a program of twelve steps to recovery. The people running the meeting really seemed to care. I was fully committed and till this day have never had a drink again.

My debt payments were overwhelming and I needed another source of income. I took a second job working as a security guard and between the two jobs was able to pay for child support, credit card bills, the union credit and a cheap car loan. After all these were paid, I had very little to live on. I gave my parents some money each month as a way of thanking them for taking me back in.

Months would sometimes pass without any problems. I was doing my best to stay on track but got frustrated at the slow pace of paying off my debt. I began to think that maybe, I could win the lottery and end my problems. I began buying lottery tickets and scratchers everyday hoping to hit the jackpot. I never did win but instead found myself going deeper in debt again. I was missing support payments as well as credit card payments and soon my days were filled with calls from creditors, my ex-wife and the credit union. I had hit financial bottom.

Through family intervention, my debts were consolidated to a single payment and the credit union negotiated a manageable payment plan so long as I stayed current with the payments. It was 1990 and I joined Gamblers Anonymous. Since joining, I have never gambled again. It took me the next 10 years before I completely paid off all of my debt.

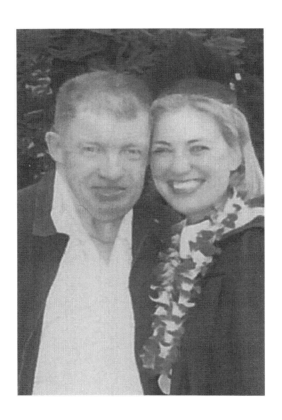

My daughter Belinda was growing to a young woman on her way to college and I could not be happier. Belinda not only graduated with a college degree, she received her Master's degree as well. It is pretty amazing to me. She is the pride and joy of my life. Despite the challenges early on in her life, she has become an accomplished woman. I could not be happier or prouder of her.

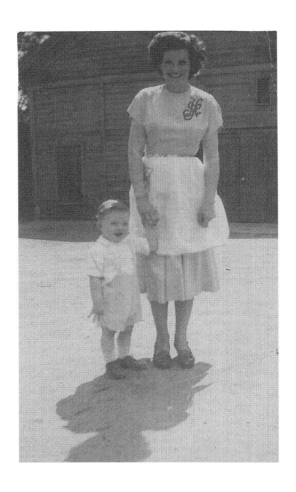

In the early 90's, as I was trying to take control of my life, I went to a veterans hospital to address a foot fungus problem that would come and go and also to find out what was causing my nerve condition. Turns out I had a common case of jungle rot and an undiagnosed problem with my nerves. They gave me crème and pills to treat my conditions. My feet would get somewhat better but my nerve problem was staying with me. They set me up with an appointment to see a psychiatrist. Why are they sending me to a shrink? I'm not imagining these problems. I really did not want to go to the appointment but then I remembered the rule, no complaining.

It was determined that I was suffering from Post Traumatic Stress Disorder. This is a physical and mental condition which would require ongoing psychiatric therapy and medication. I still did not understand what they were saying but I felt good knowing, I wasn't crazy. I was told that my condition /disability, is treatable and for my suffering, I would be compensated monetarily each month. This additional income would help me get an apartment on my own. Things were starting to get a little better financially and I hoped physically.

It was a summer Saturday morning in 1997 when I visited my parent's home and made my way to the kitchen where everyone would gather to talk while having breakfast and coffee and reading the Boston Globe. My brother noticed the thumb and index finger on my left hand was shaking and asked me why that was happening. I told him it was just my nerves acting up. Little did I know what lie ahead. This was the beginning of my illness.

At first, the trembling came and went and did not really interfere much with everyday living. The fact that the shaking would come and go, led me to believe it was something that eventually would go away. Over the next several months things pretty much stayed the same. It wasn't until about a year later that the trembling in my thumb and finger had spread to my whole left hand.

At this point, I was worried and my sister Beth took the lead in bringing me to the Beth Israel hospital for testing. I was diagnosed with early stage Parkinson's disease. I had no idea what it was and I didn't know what to think of it. I thought hadn't enough gone wrong in my life? What did I do to deserve this? I thought that God must be angry at me.

During the following year, the trembling was now beginning to show up on my right hand. It was not all the time, but it never went away for long. As the months passed, I was missing more and more work because of doctor visits. The doctors were trying to find the correct dosages of a few drugs to address my current state. During this process of experimenting, you get feeling ill sometimes because your body is rejecting certain drugs or doses. You never really stop testing because they are always adjusting your medication over your lifetime.

About a year after the original diagnosis, my left and right hands were both shaking lightly. After the second year, both forearms and hands were trembling except during the hours that my medication was at its most effective. I also began to feel muscle ache in my shoulders. My condition and my absences did not allow me to do my job any longer. The telephone company offered me a retirement package which was agreeable and welcome.

What followed sometime later was an incredibly wonderful gift given to me by my oldest sister Maryanne, a one bedroom condo that she told me I could live in as long as I wanted to. I am so thankful to her for her love. Big sisters don't come any better. What a great family I have. It brings tears to my eyes for all the love they have given me and I have for them. Each of them contributes to my life and helps make it better.

There are many other people who have made contributions to my life and you know who you are. My brother Jerry helped my daughter financially and with her academics. I love him for it. My brother Joe always has been there for me and my daughter and it was he who worked with me to stop gambling. He always gives me hope. My brother Jimmy calls me every day and is there for Belinda and I love him for this. My sister Coleen and her kid's from Seattle always send their love. Beth is my angel. If not for her care and love, I don't know where I would be. She has taken care of every detail in my life for the last 12 years. She also was there for Belinda in such a big way. God blessed me with her.

On my good days, I bring my mother the paper and coffee to her at her house. I always check in on her to make sure she is alright. At 89 she still visits me regularly and always makes me feel better. She's a great mother and I love her for it. Ed Cassidy is the older brother I never had. I'm very lucky to know him and I'm so thankful for all he does for me. What a great guy and friend.

I made a decision that I would not let this disease get in my way from the things I enjoy doing. Prayer, Alcoholics Anonymous, Gamblers Anonymous, Belinda, friends and family all gave me the strength to continue living and enjoy each day God gives me. I love to play golf with Ed and attend Alcoholics Anonymous and Gamblers Anonymous meetings. Both of these organizations helped me get thru my problems and I was determined to help others as others had helped me. There are many great people who really go out of their way to help those in need. Andy, Dave and Tommy are a few examples of these special people who go out of their way to help others in need. They have all improved my life and I am so grateful to them all.

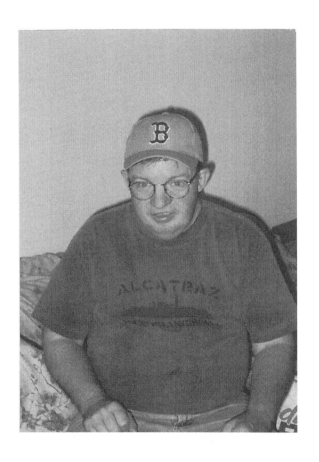

If you have a family member or a friend that has a drinking, drug or gambling problem, call these organizations for help, you may save a life. In 2010, I celebrated 27 years in Alcoholics Anonymous and 20 years in Gamblers Anonymous.

After years of paying off credit cards, union credit departments and every other kind of debt, I was finally paid off. My first action would be to help my daughter pay off her educational loans which were substantial yet worth every dollar to me. The second thing I did was buy a new golf driver. Despite my illness, I was out golfing and taking walks and even the occasional date. Some days no one could even tell I had Parkinson's. Sometimes the right medicine at the right time worked wonders. I could look at myself in the mirror and see the old me. That is what I referred to as a good day.

Five years into the illness and still swinging away and feeling good enough to travel, I went to Palm Desert, California to get away from the cold winter here in Quincy, Massachusetts. It was great seeing Jim's family and he came and stayed with me for a few days playing golf together at a couple of different times. Other than golf or eating, there seemed very little to do and I was feeling isolated and I missed my local meetings and friends. The following two years, I went to The Villages in Florida for 8 weeks and enjoyed the

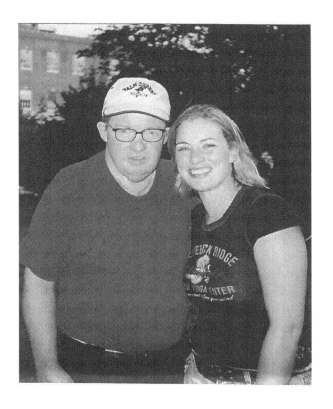

warm temperatures and other retirees who came there for the same reasons. This was an active community and I soon made a lot of friends. I tried to play often but sometimes I just ran out of strength both mentally and physically. Parkinson's doesn't take any days off. It's always there, some day's more than others. You know that you can't beat it, you just can't let it beat you.

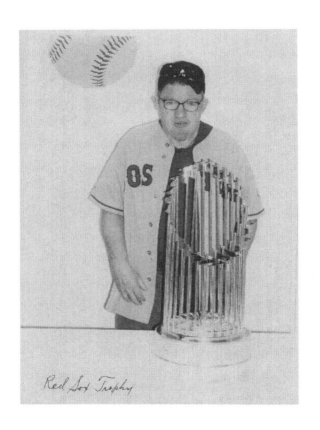

Red Sox Trophy

I noticed at times that when my four some were walking the fairways that I was falling behind the others. It seems I was taking shorter steps and I wanted to rest along the way. Remember the rule, no complaining I thought. Thank God for each day. The year was 2005 and this trip would be my last winter golfing escape.

As time passed, my illness with Parkinson's progressed. My doctor's visits increased as well. Whenever I had questions about pain in my shoulder, back, or my lack of sleep, it seemed the most common answer was "that's Parkinson's" and it probably isn't going to change. I had to learn to deal with it. That's it? That's all they can do? God, please help me with this.

After awhile, I knew that there was no magic bullet and that the doctors could only adjust my medicine. Each day was becoming a test of my will. Living alone has it's periods of loneliness but dealing with this terrible illness alone in your apartment is something else. Not only was I fighting Parkinson's but I was also dealing with what was finally diagnosed as being Post Traumatic Stress Disorder, an illness affecting the nerves and the mind.

My medications were becoming difficult to manage. Take two of these every 12 hours, one of these 3 times a day, another twice daily and one other when needed. I did my best to remember the correct times but I was slipping up or forgetting entirely. Sometimes you just forget if you took it or not.

My sister Beth, who has stood by me through this entire process, discussed my situation with the various doctor's in an attempt to make taking my medications easier and more manageable. I talk to Beth everyday and each week she comes to visit once or twice. She understands my condition better than anyone and deals directly with my doctors. It isn't easy for her because she has an important job as an attorney and is wife and mother of two small children. She travels many miles and never complains. She's always there with a big smile and a hug. I really don't know what I would do without her. I thank God that I have her. Each week she arranges my prescriptions so I won't forget to take them. I cannot tell you how many physical problems I've encountered for not taking my medications on time.

This is absolutely crucial in managing your pain and overall condition. That is why living alone with Parkinson's is so difficult. Sometimes you fall asleep and miss the time you were supposed to take your medicine. This is when Parkinson's let's go of its fury. Sometimes it is in the form of violent muscle spasms and sometimes I lose control of my legs. They just stiffen up and I'm forced to just lie there in pain for an hour or two unable to move. There are times when the pain overwhelms me and I just cry myself to sleep. This is the beast within that I deal with everyday. When you are on schedule with your meds, everything does not get all better but it is much more manageable.

By 2008, I was experiencing involuntary tongue movement. My tongue would extend itself in and out towards my lower chin .You don't even realize you are doing it .This movement also moved other muscles in my face beyond my control. Once I was traveling on a train and a little boy was sitting across from me staring at me sticking his tongue in and out. I did not realize he was copying me. Sometimes when I look in the mirror, I'm afraid of what I will see. Feeling overwhelmed at times, I cry and ask God why this is happening and could He make it stop, but there is no miracle. I've been told that God's answer comes in His time and in His way. The only hope I had, was to get some new medications that would hopefully stop this tongue activity and continue to pray for a drug to stop my shaking. When I'm going through these shaking episodes, I try to wait it out until the meds kick in. There have been times while attending an AA meeting and my shaking would come on fast and I leave hoping to get home before it peaks. Having people looking or staring at me during a shaking episode bothers me and makes me depressed. I think that they are whispering and talking about me. We all want to be seen at our best not our worst and Parkinson's is ugly to look at. It is times like these that I pray to the higher power. Everyone needs to talk to Him and he will find you. I have a grateful heart and a positive attitude which helps me get through the day.

I was told that I had an aunt who had Parkinson's and one of her symptoms was freezing up, while walking just like the Tin Man, in the Wizard of Oz ,except an oil can couldn't fix her. She had to stay in a fixed standing position for however long it took to come out of it. There is no method to the madness of this disease only that it never goes away. You may have hours of being symptom free and you learn to grab a hold of them and join the world doing the everyday things we all take granted for. I would gladly give up everything I have to be healthy again.

As the year 2009 arrived, I wanted to make this a year that I would try harder at pushing myself to exercise more and join a Parkinson's support group. I began my exercise program by walking as much as my body would allow me to. I can no longer take footsteps instead I sort of shuffle my way around with the use of a cane which I've had by my side for several years now. My condition is such that I no longer can live alone and manage my meds or household needs. Beth wanted me to move into an assisted living facility where I can get my meds given to me on schedule and all housecleaning would be performed. If needed, I can call for assistance in getting dressed, or anything else I need help with. I knew she was right, I just couldn't admit it to myself

Some days I have so much anxiety and pain that I want to scream or pound the wall with my fist. Other days, the beast sleeps. Having Parkinson's is a lot like golf. I have one good hole and one bad hole, just like the days of the week. Each day I thank my higher power for giving me a wonderful day. I also thank Him for the days that I am unable to go out, for the family and friends that call and talk to me. I have special friends like Eddie who drives me to play golf or to lunch together. My dear friend OB has passed on but his memory helps me through each day. I would not give up my life for anything. I have accepted everything that has been given to me.

Some people think I am crazy, but if all I have to do is shake and take medicine and see the doctor, then, I am all right. Though this is the hardest thing I have ever felt or had to go thru day after day, night after night, I'm able to deal with it because of my love for God. I will never abandon Him. I often speak at Alcoholics Anonymous about my difficulties and that if I can overcome my illness of alcoholism, than anyone can. I have learned so much from AA and heard other people's stories from all walks of life. We all learn to take life one day at a time, a lesson which I apply to Parkinson's.

The big day has arrived and I'm leaving Maryanne's condo to my new life at the Assisted Living house in Quincy, Massachusetts. The unknown has me both excited and cautious. The first thing I noticed when I arrived was most of the people were a lot older than me. Finding a girlfriend my age here would be tough. Most of the people seem much older than me. My apartment is beautiful with great views out the windows. I know I will be happy here. Looking around my apartment, I wonder what I did to deserve such a great place. I'm so thankful. People like myself that have Parkinson's, are always watching the clock. I have to take my meds every 3 hours of every day, every week, of every year. There is no time off. Screwing up your time schedule for meds always ends in a bad way. More pain, more depression and less movement. I was told that the nurses would come by to my apartment every three hours to remind me to take my meds and for awhile, they did. Going forward there were lapses when I overslept and the nurse never showed up. For this, I paid a steep price for being off schedule.

One time I awoke to find a nurse asleep in my room. The office people told me they would deal with the issue but I needed to be careful going forward. You can never completely trust someone else to take your meds. You either arrange a phone call or set an alarm or request a nurse. The more, the better. You're fighting a disease that never sleeps, it's always there and if you make a mistake with your meds you pay the price. Cramping muscles, violent shaking and stiffness all challenge your spirit and pain tolerance. There are times I just lie there and cry. I pray God gives me the strength to deal with my condition. This process goes on and on.

They say that Parkinson's usually affects people around 60 but I was much younger when first diagnosed. I had never heard much about Parkinson's until Michael Fox wrote a book and began speaking out about it. How he had the courage to show the world his symptoms in the hope that others would gain an understanding of what it was and his drive to fight it really impressed me. If I had one wish, it would be to talk with him and tell him that he is my hero. He helps me keep going and pushing through this disease. He is on the cutting age in treatments. He even had brain DBS surgery (deep brain surgery) to lessen his symptoms.

Unfortunately, neither surgery nor any other treatment can slow the progression of the disease but it can be helpful in improving the condition. It can reduce the medication intake which can reduce drug side effects and decrease tremors and stiffness. His surgery was on one side of the brain and Michael has said he would not have the same surgery done on the other side at this time. I guess he is looking towards new research and therapies for now.

The year is now 2010 and with the New Year comes another new symptom which is difficulty in swallowing and losing my voice for periods of time. My doctors tell me it is a fairly common symptom. My new year's resolution is not to allow this to stop my activities. Each morning that I am able, I go for a walk and depending on how I feel, I'll go to lunch with someone or attend a meeting that evening or day. I drive only when I'm shake free and not a danger to anyone or myself. Otherwise, I get a ride or stay home.

After visiting my doctor, I am taking a new medication which I'm so thankful to say has stopped my tongue movement and I'm also no longer losing my voice at least for a few weeks so far. I can go out again feeling like myself again.

There are certain things you must do every day that will help you deal with Parkinson's.

1) Try to do some kind of exercise. Walk or march in place.
2) Bend and stretch, raise your arms up and down or lift your legs when sitting down.
3) Try and keep an open mind by talking about everything else besides Parkinson's.
4) Keep your doctor's appointments.
5) THE MOST IMPORTANT ONE, TAKE YOUR MEDS ON TIME!
6) Eat properly and dress accordingly.
7) Find a support group who share your problem and support each other. You're not alone.

All of this helps. I always feel better and can do more when I've maintained these rules to live by. I have come to accept Parkinson's through God's help, my family, my friends and Michael Fox. I pray each day and ask God, did I do everything right today? I thank Him for everything I have and tell Him I never

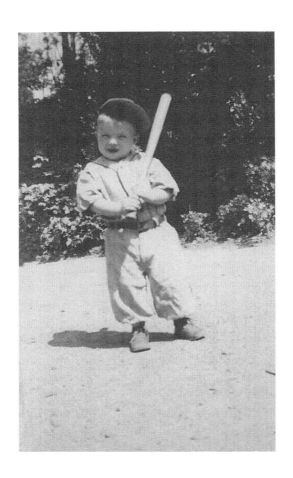

leave His side through it all. I ask for the strength to go forward and try to help others at ALCOHOLICS ANONYMOUS and GAMBLERS ANONYMOUS. I have learned that no matter how bad things in your life might seem, there is always help and people out there willing to help you. If I can do it, so can you.

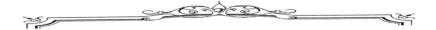

"To know Richie is to see a kind, loving man who despite his illness faces life challenges and still finds time to help others face theirs"

Love, Mom

Dad

You are my reminder that no matter how hard things get to keep going. You have changed your life for me and yourself. You are truly a role model to me and others. Through the miles, you are there for me and just call me to say I love you. You mean so much to me and I am very proud of you.

Love, Belinda

This book is the most recent testament to Richie's amazing strength of spirit that moves him to continuously strive to be all that he can be, despite enormous challenges. His embrace of a simple and profound philosophy of life is evident throughout and has been the source of great inspiration to me. I am so proud of my brother who never ceases to surprise in his endeavors and accomplishments, leads by example, gently shares his hard earned wisdom, loves with kindness and always keeps us smiling with his wonderful sense of humor. Bravo Richie!

Love, Maryanne

Richie is a strong man. He keeps people honest. And there is nothing better in this life than the freedom that comes from a true heart. We learned that from Richie. He is our hero. We love you Richie!

Love, Tom, Beth, Clara and Christopher Hurney

"As a brother Richie has always taken the time to be loving and generous, more curious about how others are doing than talking about his own trials. Now his story can be shared and we can all be inspired by this brave man with a huge heart. Congratulations Richie! Well done!"

Love, Colleen

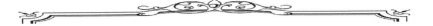

"Richie is an inspiration to us all and makes everyone he meets want to be a better person. This book, written by Rich, is a wonderful insight into true courage and the power of a loving spirit."

Love, Joe

"Richie's life has been full of challenges that he has met head on with a courageous and determined spirit. His never give up and never give in attitude is an inspiration in all who know and admire him."

Your Friend, Ed Cassidy

"Thank you for your service to your country and for reaching out to assist others in need of help. Your story truly supports the notion that anything is possible through faith, family and human intervention. Keep up the good work."

Your brother, Jim

A wise man once said "You give but a little when you give of your possessions, it is when you give of yourself that you truly give." He must have known you Richie.

Love, Maria

Made in the USA
Charleston, SC
07 July 2011